NATURAL SOLUTIONS FOR ALZHEMIER

Unlocking Cognitive Resilience For Healthy Brain, Preserving Memory, Embracing Wellness And Targeting Neural Support

DR. CARDEN KYRIE

DISCLAIMER

The only goal of this book is informational. Every effort has been taken by the author and publisher to ensure that the information provided is accurate. But the material in this book is given "as is," without any express or implied representation, warranty, or condition as to its accuracy, completeness, or suitability for any particular purpose.

Any loss, damage, or injury resulting from using the information in this book, or from any action or decision made as a result of such use, will not be covered by the author's or publisher's liability. It is recommended that readers seek the assistance of a certified specialist for guidance specific to their situation.

The opinions and viewpoints conveyed in this book belong to the author and may not necessarily represent the official stance or policies of any specified organizations or people. Any likeness to real-life occurrences, places, or people—living or deceased—is wholly coincidental.

No specific product, service, or therapy discussed in this book is endorsed by the author or publisher. Any reference to goods or services is made only for informative reasons and is not intended as a recommendation or endorsement.

Before making any judgments or acting on any information, readers are urged to independently confirm it all. Any unfavorable effects or repercussions arising from the usage of the material included in this book are disclaimed by the author and publisher.

By using this book, you consent to absolving the publisher and author of any and all claims, obligations, or losses resulting from your use of the material in it.

I appreciate your cooperation and understanding.

TABLE OF CONTENTS

CHAPTER ONE

INTRODUCTION TO ALZHEIMER

AN OVERVIEW OF ALZHEIMER'S DISEASE

Millions of people worldwide are impacted by Alzheimer's disease, a progressive neurological disease that is a major global health concern. This illness, which is characterized by memory loss, cognitive decline, and poor everyday functioning, presents significant challenges to healthcare systems, caregivers, and patients. Alzheimer's is becoming more common, especially as the population ages, and it is becoming more and more of a financial and social burden on nations. Medical research now centers on the search for efficient cures and interventions, with a focus on comprehending the underlying mechanisms and investigating various therapeutic modalities.

The etiology of Alzheimer's disease is complicated and involves the build-up of aberrant protein aggregates in the brain, including tau tangles and beta-amyloid plaques.

The steady decline in cognitive function is caused by these pathogenic alterations that interfere with neuronal connection. Alzheimer's disease is influenced by environmental and lifestyle variables as well as hereditary factors, while genetics may play a role in certain cases. The need for novel treatments becomes urgent as scientists work to understand the complex interactions between these elements.

IMPORTANCE OF HERBAL TREATMENTS

The importance of herbal medicines in the search for therapeutic options has drawn interest from the scientific community as well as from those looking for other ways to manage Alzheimer's disease. Herbal medicines are a longstanding part of traditional medicine in many different cultures. They are derived from plants and botanical sources. Studies on the neuroprotective qualities of herbs have been sparked by interest in the possible advantages of these plants in preventing cognitive decline and promoting brain health.

This emphasis on herbal cures stems from both cultural customs and an increasing understanding of the drawbacks and adverse consequences of traditional pharmaceutical therapies.

Herbal medicines have been used historically, but their relevance in the context of Alzheimer's disease goes beyond that. The potential of herbal substances to regulate oxidative stress, inflammation, and other processes linked to neurodegeneration is being closely examined. Moreover, the comprehensive character of herbal medicine, frequently incorporating an assortment of bioactive substances with possible complementary impacts, contributes a degree of intricacy to the investigation of their medicinal effectiveness. The appeal of using nature's pharmacopeia endures, even though the scientific world views these herbal medicines cautiously and acknowledges the need for thorough research and clinical validation.

The history of Alzheimer's disease highlights the urgent need for efficient treatments in light of the growing worldwide health crisis. At the same time, the investigation of herbal treatments represents a paradigm change in the treatment of cognitive diseases, acknowledging the value of natural ingredients and traditional wisdom. The junction of herbal and conventional medicines may open the door to a more all-encompassing and integrative approach to treating the intricacies of Alzheimer's Disease as research projects continue.

CHAPTER TWO

KNOWING ABOUT ALZHEIMER'S MEANING AND SIGNS

Alzheimer's disease is a neurological illness that worsens with time and mostly affects the brain, impairing memory and cognitive function. It is the most typical cause of dementia, a syndrome with a variety of symptoms that interfere with day-to-day functioning. The buildup of aberrant protein deposits in the brain, such as tau tangles and beta-amyloid plaques, which cause nerve cell death and consequent loss of cognitive function, is the defining feature of Alzheimer's disease.

Alzheimer's disease can cause a variety of symptoms, ranging in severity from memory loss and disorientation to behavioral and personality changes and trouble-solving problems. Early on, people may have occasional confusion and minor amnesia, but as the illness advances, these symptoms get worse and interfere with a person's capacity to carry out daily activities on their own. The disease is made more complex by the behavioral and psychological symptoms that frequently coexist with cognitive impairment, such as aggressiveness, agitation, and mood swings.

REASONS AND DANGER ELEMENTS

Although the precise origins of Alzheimer's disease are still unknown, a mix of lifestyle, environmental, and genetic variables are thought to play a role in the disease's development. Alzheimer's risk can be raised by genetic predisposition, especially if specific genes, such as Apolipoprotein E (APOE), are present. Furthermore, risk factors include age, family history, and a few medical disorders like diabetes and cardiovascular disease. Additionally, recent studies point to a connection between oxidative stress, chronic inflammation, and the onset of Alzheimer's disease.

ALZHEIMER'S DISEASE STAGES

Alzheimer's disease develops in phases, each of which has unique functional and cognitive alterations. People may have slight cognitive impairment and minor memory lapses in the early stages. Memory loss intensifies as the disease progresses to the moderate stage, and people may find it difficult to do daily activities like eating and dressing. People lose their capacity for basic self-care, communication, and recognition of loved ones during the severe stage. Each person's experience with Alzheimer's disease is unique, as is the length of time each stage lasts.

CURRENT METHODS OF TREATMENT

Alzheimer's disease currently has no known cure; instead, care aims to manage symptoms and enhance the quality of life for those who are afflicted. Cholinesterase inhibitors (donepezil, rivastigmine) and memantine are examples of medications that may be used to treat cognitive problems and control neurotransmitters in the brain. A treatment plan must also include non-pharmacological therapies including social interaction, physical activity, and cognitive stimulation. Support and education for caregivers are essential in assisting families in overcoming the difficulties brought on by Alzheimer's disease and guaranteeing the well-being of both the affected person and their carers.

Alzheimer's disease is a crippling and complicated illness that has a significant effect on both the affected person and their family. Comprehending the disease's definition, signs, causes, and phases is essential for prompt diagnosis and efficient treatment. Current approaches to treatment focus on symptom relief and improving overall quality of life, but more research is needed to understand the underlying mechanisms of Alzheimer's and create specific medicines to address the disease's underlying causes.

CHAPTER THREE

PRINCIPLES AND PRACTICES OF HERBALISM

OVERVIEW OF HERBAL MEDICINE

Using plants and plant extracts to treat a variety of illnesses, herbal medicine also referred to as phytotherapy or botanical medicine is an age-old kind of alternative medicine. This age-old method has strong cultural origins, and the evolution of medical procedures has been greatly aided by the use of herbal treatments. Enlisting the help of plant chemicals like flavonoids, alkaloids, and essential oils to enhance the body's inherent healing abilities is the cornerstone of herbal therapy.

Plants with a wide variety of therapeutic qualities are included in herbal medicine. Herbalism's holistic approach recognizes the connection between the environment, the mind, and the body. Herbal medicine practitioners frequently stress the value of customized treatment regimens that consider the patient's general health in addition to their symptoms.

This individualized approach is consistent with the theory that every individual reacts differently to herbal medicines and that a variety of factors, including heredity, lifestyle, and constitution, can affect how effective a therapy is.

SAFETY CONSIDERATIONS

Although herbal therapy provides a natural and comprehensive approach to health, it is important to understand that not all herbs are suitable for all individuals or circumstances. Knowing the possible hazards and contraindications related to particular plants is important for safety concerns while using herbal remedies. Some medical conditions, drugs, or pregnancy may have negative interactions with specific plants.

Before adding herbal medicines to their wellness regimens, people should always speak with licensed herbalists or healthcare experts, especially if they are using prescription medications or have pre-existing health concerns.

Ensuring safety also involves quality control and herb sourcing. Plant identity errors, contamination, or inadequate processing might jeopardize the effectiveness and security of herbal products. For this reason, it's critical to get herbs from reliable suppliers and follow dose recommendations.

Promoting safe herbal practices requires education because it equips people with the knowledge necessary to make informed decisions about their health by letting them know about possible interactions and side effects.

HERBAL FORMULATIONS AND DOSES

To create remedies that specifically address health concerns, different plant extracts are combined in herbal formulations. A thorough understanding of the characteristics and interactions between various herbs is essential to the art and science of creating herbal remedies. Herbalists evaluate aspects such as the plant's active ingredients, its traditional uses, and the desired medicinal outcome when developing formulations. Tinctures, teas, capsules, and topical preparations are common forms of herbal formulations, each offering unique benefits and absorption profiles.

Dosages in herbal medicine are not one-size-fits-all and depend on various factors, including the individual's age, weight, and the severity of the condition being treated. Herbalists often employ a titration approach, gradually adjusting dosages to observe the body's response. This cautious method minimizes the risk of adverse reactions while allowing for personalized treatment.

The integration of herbal medicine into mainstream healthcare often involves collaboration between herbalists and conventional healthcare providers to establish optimal dosages and ensure safe coadministration with other treatments.

INTERACTIONS WITH CONVENTIONAL MEDICATIONS

Understanding the potential interactions between herbal remedies and conventional medications is imperative for ensuring the safety and efficacy of combined treatments. Certain herbs may enhance or inhibit the effects of pharmaceutical drugs, leading to unpredictable outcomes. For example, herbs with anticoagulant properties may interact with blood-thinning medications, potentially increasing the risk of bleeding. Communication between healthcare professionals and patients about their use of herbal supplements is crucial, as it allows for the identification of potential interactions and the adjustment of treatment plans accordingly.

The complex nature of herb-drug interactions underscores the importance of an integrative approach to healthcare. Collaboration between herbalists and conventional healthcare providers enables a comprehensive understanding of the patient's health profile, leading to more informed decisions about treatment strategies. Additionally, research efforts aimed at elucidating herb-drug interactions contribute to the growing body of knowledge that guides both herbalists and medical practitioners in delivering safe and effective care.

CHAPTER FOUR

KEY HERBS FOR COGNITIVE HEALTH

GINKGO BILOBA

Ginkgo Biloba is a well-known herb that has been used for centuries in traditional medicine, particularly in Chinese and Japanese practices. The leaves of the Ginkgo tree are rich in flavonoids and terpenoids, which are believed to have antioxidant properties. These antioxidants may help protect the cells of the brain from oxidative stress, potentially reducing the risk of cognitive decline.

Ginkgo Biloba is often touted for its ability to improve blood flow, including to the brain, which is crucial for optimal cognitive function. Some studies suggest that Ginkgo Biloba may be beneficial for conditions like age-related cognitive decline and mild memory impairment.

TURMERIC AND CURCUMIN

Turmeric and its active compound, Curcumin, have gained significant attention for their potential cognitive health benefits. Turmeric, a bright yellow spice commonly used in Indian cuisine, has anti-inflammatory and antioxidant properties. Curcumin, the key bioactive component in turmeric, has been studied for its potential neuroprotective effects. It may cross the blood-brain barrier and has been shown to possess anti-inflammatory and antioxidant properties, which could contribute to cognitive health. Some research suggests that Curcumin may play a role in the prevention or management of neurodegenerative diseases, such as Alzheimer's.

SAGE

Sage, a fragrant herb with a long history of culinary and medicinal use, is believed to have cognitive-enhancing properties. It contains compounds like rosmarinic acid, which has antioxidant and anti-inflammatory effects.

Sage has been traditionally used to enhance memory and concentration, and some studies suggest that it may have potential benefits for cognitive function. While more research is needed to fully understand the mechanisms behind these effects, incorporating sage into the diet or using it as a supplement is a practice that aligns with the traditional uses of this herb for cognitive well-being.

ROSEMARY

Rosemary is another herb with a rich history of culinary and medicinal use, and it is often associated with memory enhancement. The aroma of rosemary has been linked to improved cognitive performance and mood. Rosemary contains compounds like ursolic acid and rosmarinic acid, which may have neuroprotective effects. Some studies suggest that inhaling the scent of rosemary essential oil may lead to improvements in memory and alertness. Additionally, rosemary extract has demonstrated antioxidant and anti-inflammatory properties, which could contribute to its potential cognitive health benefits.

HUPERZINE A

Huperzine A, derived from a type of club moss (Huperzia serrata), is a natural compound that has been investigated for its potential cognitive-enhancing effects. It is known to inhibit acetylcholinesterase, an enzyme that breaks down acetylcholine, a neurotransmitter involved in learning and memory. Huperzine A may raise acetylcholine levels by blocking this enzyme, which could enhance cognitive function. Some studies suggest that Huperzine A may be beneficial for conditions like Alzheimer's disease and age-related cognitive decline. However, more research is needed to establish its long-term safety and efficacy.

These key herbs Ginkgo Biloba, Turmeric and Curcumin, Sage, Rosemary, and Huperzine A have been studied for their potential cognitive health benefits. While some research supports their positive effects on memory, concentration, and overall brain function, it's important to note that individual responses may vary. Integrating these herbs into a balanced and varied diet, in consultation with a healthcare professional, may offer a natural approach to supporting cognitive well-being. However, more rigorous research is needed to fully understand the mechanisms and long-term effects of these herbs on cognitive health.

CHAPTER FIVE

HERBAL WAYS OF LIVING

NUTRITIONAL POINTS TO REMEMBER

When it comes to Herbal Lifestyle Practices, nutrition is a critical factor in fostering general health. To promote the body's natural processes, traditional herbal wisdom frequently emphasizes the ingestion of foods and herbs high in nutrients. It is thought that a diet high in a variety of plant-based foods, such as fruits, vegetables, and whole grains, provides vital vitamins and minerals that support good health. To maximize particular health benefits, herbal supplements like adaptogenic herbs and medicinal plants are often incorporated into dietary regimens. By utilizing the medicinal qualities of different herbs, this all-encompassing approach to diet seeks to both nourish the body and address specific health issues for each individual.

MENTAL WORKOUTS

Key components of the Herbal Lifestyle Practices, which emphasize the comprehensive development of mental abilities, are cognitive exercises. The purpose of these exercises is to improve cognitive abilities such as problem-solving, memory, and attention. Herbal medicines are frequently used to support cognitive health, such as Bacopa monnieri and Ginkgo biloba. Herbal teas like chamomile or lavender, as well as meditation and mindfulness exercises, are popular because of their relaxing properties that promote emotional and mental clarity. As part of their holistic herbal lifestyle, people seek to maintain cognitive sharpness and improve mental resilience by combining cognitive activities with herbal interventions.

TECHNIQUES FOR STRESS MANAGEMENT

A key component of herbal lifestyle practices is effective stress management, which acknowledges the complex relationship between the mind and body. Herbal therapies that modulate the body's stress response include adaptogenic herbs (Rhodiola rosea, ashwagandha, etc.). Mind-body practices, such as yoga and tai chi, are popular because they have a positive effect on both stress relief and physical health. Incorporating herbal teas, such as passionflower or holy basil, also offers a calming routine that helps reduce stress. Herbal practices' comprehensive approach to stress management places a strong emphasis on modifying one's lifestyle, practicing mindfulness, and incorporating adaptogenic herbs to strengthen one's resistance to the stresses of contemporary life.

SUITABLE SLEEP POSITION

According to the Herbal Lifestyle Practices, good sleep hygiene is essential for general health and well-being. Herbal treatments with soothing characteristics, such as chamomile and valerian root, are used to promote relaxation and enhance the quality of sleep. Herbal remedies for encouraging sound sleep are enhanced by creating a sleep-friendly atmosphere that includes herbal essential oils like lavender. Sleep hygiene is a crucial part of the herbal lifestyle, and practices like setting up nighttime routines and minimizing screen time before bed are essential. People who are aware of the significant effects that good sleep has on their physical and mental well-being try to enhance their sleep patterns by integrating herbal therapies with mindful sleep techniques.

CHAPTER SIX

HERBAL TREATMENTS IN CONVENTIONAL MEDICINE

CHINESE TRADITIONAL MEDICINE

The foundational ideas of traditional Chinese medicine (TCM), which has a storied 2,000-year history, are based on a holistic view of health and wellbeing. The core tenet of TCM is the idea that qi, or life force, flows and balances throughout the body. To keep the body in balance, this age-old method combines acupuncture, massage, herbal medicines, and food regimens.

GINSENG

An important role for the well-known TCM herb ginseng played in conventional medical procedures. The adaptogenic qualities of Panax ginseng, often known as Asian or Korean ginseng, are widely prized. Ginseng is a common herb used by TCM practitioners to boost vitality overall, increase energy levels, and fortify the body's resistance to stress. The ginseng plant's root is thought to help qi return to equilibrium, enhancing longevity and general well-being.

KOLA GOTU

Another herb with a long history of use in traditional medicine is gotu kola, which has been used for ages in many Asan cultures. Gotu Kola, also called Centella Asiatica, is highly valued for its possible advantages to the circulatory and cognitive systems. According to Traditional Chinese Medicine (TCM), gotu kola is a herb that supports good blood circulation and fosters mental clarity while also nourishing the body. It is frequently included in herbal remedies to treat inflammatory diseases and improve cognitive performance in general.

CHINESE CLUB MOSS

Chinese club moss, or Huperzia serrata in scientific parlance, is a herb used in traditional Chinese medicine to promote mental well-being. In TCM, huperzine A, the main ingredient, is frequently used to treat disorders related to memory and cognitive loss because it is thought to have neuroprotective properties. Chinese Club Moss may be suggested by TCM practitioners as part of a comprehensive strategy to support brain function and preserve mental sharpness.

In Traditional Chinese Medicine (TCM), the choice of herbs is determined by both their unique qualities and how well they work together in herbal compositions. It is believed that the combination of herbs will improve therapeutic results and address imbalances more thoroughly. TCM practitioners develop individualized remedies to reestablish the body's equilibrium, taking into account the patient's constitution, the unique characteristics of the illness, and the interactions between various herbs.

While TCM has a long history of use and many people attest to its usefulness, it is crucial to remember that herbal treatments should be used cautiously. It is best to seek advice from a licensed Traditional Chinese Medicine practitioner to make sure that the herbs selected are appropriate for each person's specific medical needs. Furthermore, including herbal treatments into one's regimen should be done under a healthcare provider's supervision and with awareness of any potential drug interactions.

AYURVEDIC HEALTH CARE

The traditional medical practice of Ayurveda, which has its roots in ancient India, is based on the idea that equilibrium is necessary for good health. According to Ayurveda, the human body is an intricate combination of the vata, pitta, and kapha doshas, or three basic energies. It is thought that every individual has a distinct constitution, or Prakriti, that defines their physical and mental qualities. By taking into account a person's Prakriti and how outside influences affect their general health, Ayurvedic practitioners seek to bring their body back into harmony.

ASHWAGANDHA

Ashwagandha (Withania somnifera), a well-known plant in Ayurvedic medicine, is prized for its adaptogenic qualities. It's well known that ashwagandha fosters resilience and aids in the body's adjustment to stress. It is frequently used to support the neurological system, increase vigor, and strengthen the immunological system. This plant is also known for its ability to enhance cognitive performance and lessen depressive and anxious symptoms. Common forms of ashwagandha consumption include powders, pills, and supplements used in Ayurvedic formulas.

BACOPA MONNIERI, OR BRAHMI

Another important herb in Ayurveda is Brahmi (Bacopa monnieri), which is renowned for its ability to improve cognition. Traditionally used to boost memory, focus, and overall brain function, Brahmi is also referred to as water hyssop. It is useful in Ayurvedic formulations meant to support mental clarity and focus because it is said to have a relaxing impact on the mind. To maximize its possible cognitive benefits, Brahmi is commonly taken as herbal teas, extracts, or supplements.

SACRED BASIL (TULSI)

In Ayurvedic medicine, holy basil, also known as Tulsi (Ocimum sanctum), is highly valued for its all-encompassing therapeutic abilities. Tulsi is regarded as an adaptogen, assisting the body in preserving equilibrium and managing stress. It is well-known for having antioxidant, anti-inflammatory, and antibacterial qualities. Common uses for tulsi include immune system support, cold and cough relief, and respiratory health promotion. It is also prized for its capacity to improve digestion and promote general health. To make use of its many health advantages, tulsi is frequently drunk as tea or added to Ayurvedic formulas.

Ayurvedic medicine emphasizes the restoration of equilibrium in both the body and the mind, encapsulating a holistic approach to health. Holy basil, ashwagandha, and Brahmi represent the long history of herbal medicines in Ayurveda, providing a holistic approach to health that has lasted for centuries. These herbs embody the holistic approach of Ayurvedic medicine by promoting mental and emotional balance as well as physical health, as well as the complex relationship between the two.

CHAPTER SEVEN

COMBINING TRADITIONAL MEDICAL CARE WITH HERBAL REMEDIES

WORKING TOGETHER

Combining the advantages of traditional and modern healthcare methods calls for a cooperative approach when integrating herbal treatments with conventional treatment. To guarantee patient well-being and maximize therapeutic results, this synergy is crucial. To develop a thorough and all-encompassing healthcare plan, collaborative approaches highlight the significance of communication and cooperation between patients, medical experts, and herbal practitioners.

SPEAKING WITH MEDICAL EXPERTS

A vital stage in the integration process is consulting with medical experts. It is recommended that patients inform their healthcare professionals about their usage of herbal treatments to promote candid and educated dialogue. Assessing the possible interactions between herbal medicines and conventional medications is a crucial task for healthcare providers. This cooperative consultation aids in risk minimization, identification of any contraindications, and confirmation that the patient's health objectives are in line with the treatment plan as a whole.

RESEARCH RESULTS AND CLINICAL TRIALS

Evidence-based herbal remedy integration with conventional treatment is based on clinical trials and research findings. Thorough scientific research yields important information on the safety, effectiveness, and possible adverse effects of herbal remedies. When prescribing or including herbal treatments in a treatment plan, medical professionals can make well-informed decisions when these findings are incorporated into clinical practice. In addition, continual research helps integrated approaches remain better over time, guaranteeing that patients receive the best possible therapy that is supported by evidence.

The cooperative strategy creates a forum for knowledge and experience sharing between herbalists and medical professionals. There is no one-size-fits-all strategy for incorporating herbal treatments into conventional treatment approaches; instead, patient-centered, individualized care is needed. The collaborative model facilitates the exchange of expertise, guaranteeing that the integration process is customized to meet the specific needs of each patient, accounting for variables like lifestyle, preferences, and medical history.

It's important to integrate herbal medicines with caution, even with their potential benefits. Some issues must be properly handled, including the lack of defined dosing, quality control, and possible interactions with pharmaceutical medications. A collaborative approach's essential elements include clinical monitoring and routine follow-ups, which enable medical personnel to evaluate the patient's reaction to the integrated treatment and make any required modifications.

The process of integrating herbal treatments with conventional treatment is dynamic and collaborative, necessitating open communication, professional consultation with healthcare providers, and reliance on research findings and clinical trials. An all-encompassing, patient-centered strategy that promotes the best possible health outcomes and guarantees the safety and effectiveness of the integrated treatment plan can be formed by fusing the best aspects of modern and traditional healthcare.

CHAPTER EIGHT

SAFETY MEASURES AND POSSIBLE ADVERSE REACTIONS

SENSITIVITIES AND ALLERGIES

The risk of allergies and sensitivities is one of the most important things to take into account when using herbs or herbal medicines. Some people may have previously experienced allergic reactions to particular plants, herbs, or their constituent parts. Skin rashes, itching, swelling, respiratory discomfort, and digestive problems are just a few of the ways that allergic reactions can present themselves. Before adding any new herbs to their wellness routines, people must be fully informed of their allergies and sensitivities.

Additionally, cross-reactivity is an important consideration. Some people could be sensitive to a specific plant or herb because they share allergies with other things, such as foods or environmental allergens. Therefore, if there is any doubt regarding possible cross-reactivity, it is advised to proceed with caution, carry out in-depth research, or speak with a healthcare provider.

APPROPRIATE OBSERVATION

Even though herbal medicines are frequently seen as natural and secure, it is crucial to stress the significance of appropriate supervision when using them. Herbal remedies may have varying effects on each person, and the results might be influenced by age, pre-existing medical issues, and drug combinations. It is essential to regularly monitor one's health and any changes in symptoms to evaluate the safety and efficacy of the herbal medicine.

It is advised to begin with modest herb dosages and monitor any reactions or adverse effects. Depending on each person's reaction, alterations to the dosage or stopping altogether can be required. Additionally, since possible interactions may affect the safety and effectiveness of both therapies, monitoring is even more important when using herbal medicines in addition to conventional pharmaceuticals. It is essential to have regular contact with a healthcare provider to guarantee appropriate monitoring and quickly address any concerns.

WHEN NOT TO USE A PARTICULAR HERB:

Even though herbs are generally seen to be harmless, there are several situations in which they should not be used. For example, those who are pregnant or nursing should use caution and consult with healthcare professionals before using any particular herb because it may not be well-established that it is safe to use at these times. Likewise, people who already have health issues, such as liver or renal problems, might need to stay away from certain herbs because they might make their diseases worse.

Moreover, some herbs have the potential to interact negatively with pharmaceuticals, resulting in side effects or decreased effectiveness. Before adding herbs to a treatment plan, it is important to be aware of any contraindications and speak with medical authorities, especially if you are on prescription medications.

Ethical herbal use requires a thorough understanding of allergies and sensitivities, appropriate monitoring, and knowledge of when to avoid particular herbs. Through a focus on safety and specific health considerations, people can maximize the potential advantages of herbal treatments while reducing the hazards that come with using them. Before starting any herbal regimen, always get the advice of a licensed healthcare provider, especially if you have any questions or concerns.

CHAPTER NINE

HERBAL WAYS OF LIVING

NUTRITIONAL POINTS TO REMEMBER

When it comes to Herbal Lifestyle Practices, nutrition is a critical factor in fostering general health. To promote the body's natural processes, traditional herbal wisdom frequently emphasizes the ingestion of foods and herbs high in nutrients. It is thought that a diet high in a variety of plant-based foods, such as fruits, vegetables, and whole grains, provides vital vitamins and minerals that support good health. To maximize particular health benefits, herbal supplements like adaptogenic herbs and medicinal plants are often incorporated into dietary regimens. By utilizing the medicinal qualities of different herbs, this all-encompassing approach to diet seeks to both nourish the body and address specific health issues for each individual.

MENTAL WORKOUTS

Key components of the Herbal Lifestyle Practices, which emphasize the comprehensive development of mental abilities, are cognitive exercises. The purpose of these exercises is to improve cognitive abilities such as problem-solving, memory, and attention. Herbal medicines are frequently used to support cognitive health, such as Bacopa monnieri and Ginkgo biloba. Herbal teas like chamomile or lavender, as well as meditation and mindfulness exercises, are popular because of their relaxing properties that promote emotional and mental clarity. As part of their holistic herbal lifestyle, people seek to maintain cognitive sharpness and improve mental resilience by combining cognitive activities with herbal interventions.

TECHNIQUES FOR STRESS MANAGEMENT

A key component of herbal lifestyle practices is effective stress management, which acknowledges the complex relationship between the mind and body. Herbal therapies that modulate the body's stress response include adaptogenic herbs (Rhodiola rosea, ashwagandha, etc.). Mind-body practices, such as yoga and tai chi, are popular because they have a positive effect on both stress relief and physical health. Incorporating herbal teas, such as passionflower or holy basil, also offers a calming routine that helps reduce stress. Herbal practices' comprehensive approach to stress management places a strong emphasis on modifying one's lifestyle, practicing mindfulness, and incorporating adaptogenic herbs to strengthen one's resistance to the stresses of contemporary life.

SUITABLE SLEEP POSITION

According to the Herbal Lifestyle Practices, good sleep hygiene is essential for general health and well-being. Herbal treatments with soothing characteristics, such as chamomile and valerian root, are used to promote relaxation and enhance the quality of sleep. Herbal remedies for encouraging sound sleep are enhanced by creating a sleep-friendly atmosphere that includes herbal essential oils like lavender. Sleep hygiene is a crucial part of the herbal lifestyle, and practices like setting up nighttime routines and minimizing screen time before bed are essential. People who are aware of the significant effects that good sleep has on their physical and mental well-being try to enhance their sleep patterns by integrating herbal therapies with mindful sleep techniques.

CHAPTER TEN

HERBAL TREATMENTS IN CONVENTIONAL MEDICINE

CHINESE TRADITIONAL MEDICINE

The foundational ideas of traditional Chinese medicine (TCM), which has a storied 2,000-year history, are based on a holistic view of health and wellbeing. The core tenet of TCM is the idea that qi, or life force, flows and balances throughout the body. To keep the body in balance, this age-old method combines acupuncture, massage, herbal medicines, and food regimens.

GINSENG

An important role for the well-known TCM herb ginseng played in conventional medical procedures. The adaptogenic qualities of Panax ginseng, often known as Asian or Korean ginseng, are widely prized. Ginseng is a common herb used by TCM practitioners to boost vitality overall, increase energy levels, and fortify the body's resistance to stress. The ginseng plant's root is thought to help qi return to equilibrium, enhancing longevity and general well-being.

KOLA GOTU

Another herb with a long history of use in traditional medicine is gotu kola, which has been used for ages in many Asan cultures. Gotu Kola, also called Centella Asiatica, is highly valued for its possible advantages to the circulatory and cognitive systems. According to Traditional Chinese Medicine (TCM), gotu kola is a herb that supports good blood circulation and fosters mental clarity while also nourishing the body. It is frequently included in herbal remedies to treat inflammatory diseases and improve cognitive performance in general.

CHINESE CLUB MOSS

Chinese club moss, or Huperzia serrata in scientific parlance, is a herb used in traditional Chinese medicine to promote mental well-being. In TCM, huperzine A, the main ingredient, is frequently used to treat disorders related to memory and cognitive loss because it is thought to have neuroprotective properties. Chinese Club Moss may be suggested by TCM practitioners as part of a comprehensive strategy to support brain function and preserve mental sharpness.

In Traditional Chinese Medicine (TCM), the choice of herbs is determined by both their unique qualities and how well they work together in herbal compositions. It is believed that the combination of herbs will improve therapeutic results and address imbalances more thoroughly. TCM practitioners develop individualized remedies to reestablish the body's equilibrium, taking into account the patient's constitution, the unique characteristics of the illness, and the interactions between various herbs.

While TCM has a long history of use and many people attest to its usefulness, it is crucial to remember that herbal treatments should be used cautiously. It is best to seek advice from a licensed Traditional Chinese Medicine practitioner to make sure that the herbs selected are appropriate for each person's specific medical needs. Furthermore, including herbal treatments into one's regimen should be done under a healthcare provider's supervision and with awareness of any potential drug interactions.

AYURVEDIC HEALTH CARE

The traditional medical practice of Ayurveda, which has its roots in ancient India, is based on the idea that equilibrium is necessary for good health. According to Ayurveda, the human body is an intricate combination of the vata, pitta, and kapha doshas, or three basic energies. It is thought that every individual has a distinct constitution, or Prakriti, that defines their physical and mental qualities. By taking into account a person's Prakriti and how outside influences affect their general health, Ayurvedic practitioners seek to bring their body back into harmony.

ASHWAGANDHA

Ashwagandha (Withania somnifera), a well-known plant in Ayurvedic medicine, is prized for its adaptogenic qualities. It's well known that ashwagandha fosters resilience and aids in the body's adjustment to stress. It is frequently used to support the neurological system, increase vigor, and strengthen the immunological system. This plant is also known for its ability to enhance cognitive performance and lessen depressive and anxious symptoms. Common forms of ashwagandha consumption include powders, pills, and supplements used in Ayurvedic formulas.

BACOPA MONNIERI, OR BRAHMI

Another important herb in Ayurveda is Brahmi (Bacopa monnieri), which is renowned for its ability to improve cognition. Traditionally used to boost memory, focus, and overall brain function, Brahmi is also referred to as water hyssop. It is useful in Ayurvedic formulations meant to support mental clarity and focus because it is said to have a relaxing impact on the mind. To maximize its possible cognitive benefits, Brahmi is commonly taken as herbal teas, extracts, or supplements.

SACRED BASIL (TULSI)

In Ayurvedic medicine, holy basil, also known as Tulsi (Ocimum sanctum), is highly valued for its all-encompassing therapeutic abilities. Tulsi is regarded as an adaptogen, assisting the body in preserving equilibrium and managing stress. It is well-known for having antioxidant, anti-inflammatory, and antibacterial qualities. Common uses for tulsi include immune system support, cold and cough relief, and respiratory health promotion. It is also prized for its capacity to improve digestion and promote general health. To make use of its many health advantages, tulsi is frequently drunk as tea or added to Ayurvedic formulas.

CHAPTER ELEVEN

COMBINING TRADITIONAL MEDICAL CARE WITH HERBAL REMEDIES

WORKING TOGETHER

Combining the advantages of traditional and modern healthcare methods calls for a cooperative approach when integrating herbal treatments with conventional treatment. To guarantee patient well-being and maximize therapeutic results, this synergy is crucial. To develop a thorough and all-encompassing healthcare plan, collaborative approaches highlight the significance of communication and cooperation between patients, medical experts, and herbal practitioners.

SPEAKING WITH MEDICAL EXPERTS

A vital stage in the integration process is consulting with medical experts. It is recommended that patients inform their healthcare professionals about their usage of herbal treatments to promote candid and educated dialogue. Assessing the possible interactions between herbal medicines and conventional medications is a crucial task for healthcare providers. This cooperative consultation aids in risk minimization, identification of any contraindications, and confirmation that the patient's health objectives are in line with the treatment plan as a whole.

RESEARCH RESULTS AND CLINICAL TRIALS

Evidence-based herbal remedy integration with conventional treatment is based on clinical trials and research findings. Thorough scientific research yields important information on the safety, effectiveness, and possible adverse effects of herbal remedies. When prescribing or including herbal treatments in a treatment plan, medical professionals can make well-informed decisions when these findings are incorporated into clinical practice. In addition, continual research helps integrated approaches remain better over time, guaranteeing that patients receive the best possible therapy that is supported by evidence.

The cooperative strategy creates a forum for knowledge and experience sharing between herbalists and medical professionals. There is no one-size-fits-all strategy for incorporating herbal treatments into conventional treatment approaches; instead, patient-centered, individualized care is needed. The collaborative model facilitates the exchange of expertise, guaranteeing that the integration process is customized to meet the specific needs of each patient, accounting for variables like lifestyle, preferences, and medical history.

It's important to integrate herbal medicines with caution, even with their potential benefits. Some issues must be properly handled, including the lack of defined dosing, quality control, and possible interactions with pharmaceutical medications. A collaborative approach's essential elements include clinical monitoring and routine follow-ups, which enable medical personnel to evaluate the patient's reaction to the integrated treatment and make any required modifications.

The process of integrating herbal treatments with conventional treatment is dynamic and collaborative, necessitating open communication, professional consultation with healthcare providers, and reliance on research findings and clinical trials. An all-encompassing, patient-centered strategy that promotes the best possible health outcomes and guarantees the safety and effectiveness of the integrated treatment plan can be formed by fusing the best aspects of modern and traditional healthcare.

CHAPTER TWELVE

SAFETY MEASURES AND POSSIBLE ADVERSE REACTIONS

SENSITIVITIES AND ALLERGIES

The risk of allergies and sensitivities is one of the most important things to take into account when using herbs or herbal medicines. Some people may have previously experienced allergic reactions to particular plants, herbs, or their constituent parts. Skin rashes, itching, swelling, respiratory discomfort, and digestive problems are just a few of the ways that allergic reactions can present themselves. Before adding any new herbs to their wellness routines, people must be fully informed of their allergies and sensitivities.

Additionally, cross-reactivity is an important consideration. Some people could be sensitive to a specific plant or herb because they share allergies with other things, such as foods or environmental allergens. Therefore, if there is any doubt regarding possible cross-reactivity, it is advised to proceed with caution, carry out in-depth research, or speak with a healthcare provider.

APPROPRIATE OBSERVATION

Even though herbal medicines are frequently seen as natural and secure, it is crucial to stress the significance of appropriate supervision when using them. Herbal remedies may have varying effects on each person, and the results might be influenced by age, pre-existing medical issues, and drug combinations. It is essential to regularly monitor one's health and any changes in symptoms to evaluate the safety and efficacy of the herbal medicine.

It is advised to begin with modest herb dosages and monitors any reactions or adverse effects. Depending on each person's reaction, alterations to the dosage or stopping altogether can be required. Additionally, since possible interactions may affect the safety and effectiveness of both therapies, monitoring is even more important when using herbal medicines in addition to conventional pharmaceuticals. It is essential to have regular contact with a healthcare provider to guarantee appropriate monitoring and quickly address any concerns.

WHEN NOT TO USE A PARTICULAR HERB:

Even though herbs are generally seen to be harmless, there are several situations in which they should not be used. For example, those who are pregnant or nursing should use caution and consult with healthcare professionals before using any particular herb because it may not be well-established that it is safe to use at these times. Likewise, people who already have health issues, such as liver or renal problems, might need to stay away from certain herbs because they might make their diseases worse.

Moreover, some herbs have the potential to interact negatively with pharmaceuticals, resulting in side effects or decreased effectiveness. Before adding herbs to a treatment plan, it is important to be aware of any contraindications and speak with medical authorities, especially if you are on prescription medications.

Ethical herbal use requires a thorough understanding of allergies and sensitivities, appropriate monitoring, and knowledge of when to avoid particular herbs. Through a focus on safety and specific health considerations, people can maximize the potential advantages of herbal treatments while reducing the hazards that come with using them. Before starting any herbal regimen, always get the advice of a licensed healthcare provider, especially if you have any questions or concerns.